AF306524

François KALENGA LUHEMBWE
Michel KABAMBA NZAJI

Risk factors for low birth weight

François KALENGA LUHEMBWE
Michel KABAMBA NZAJI

Risk factors for low birth weight

Kamina, DRCongo

Imprint

Any brand names and product names mentioned in this book are subject to trademark, brand or patent protection and are trademarks or registered trademarks of their respective holders. The use of brand names, product names, common names, trade names, product descriptions etc. even without a particular marking in this work is in no way to be construed to mean that such names may be regarded as unrestricted in respect of trademark and brand protection legislation and could thus be used by anyone.

Cover image: www.ingimage.com

This book is a translation from the original published under ISBN 978-620-6-70956-5.

Publisher:
Sciencia Scripts
is a trademark of
Dodo Books Indian Ocean Ltd. and OmniScriptum S.R.L publishing group

120 High Road, East Finchley, London, N2 9ED, United Kingdom
Str. Armeneasca 28/1, office 1, Chisinau MD-2012, Republic of Moldova, Europe
Printed at: see last page
ISBN: 978-620-8-11265-3

TABLE OF

SUMMARY

Introduction: Because of its impact on infant morbidity and mortality, and its implications for adult health, low birth weight is a major public health problem in the DRC. The present study was carried out at the Kamina general referral hospital, with the objectives of determining the frequency of LBW in the Kamina health zone and identifying the various factors that may be associated with it.

Methodology: This is a case-control study nested within a cross-sectional study that included live and non-living births registered at HGR/Kamina from December 2022 to July 2023. The Pearson Chi-Square test was used to test for dependence between FPN (dependent variable) and the other independent variables. The significance level is set at a value of $P<0.05$. The Odds ratio (OR) and its 95% confidence interval (95% CI) were calculated to determine the association between the random variables. Logistic regression using Wald's stepwise method was used to adjust the Odds Ratio.

Results: The frequency of LBW in our study setting was 14.28%. Risk factors for low birth weight were unwanted pregnancy (ORa=32.736 ; IC95%= [3.361-318.829] ; pa=0.003) , hospitalization during pregnancy (ORa=179.877 ; CI95%= [10.354-10.354]; pa=0.00) and passive smoking by the mother during pregnancy (ORa=35.869; CI95%= [2.807-458.398]; pa=0.006).

Conclusion: This study has shown that, in addition to non-modifiable physiological determinants, certain important determinants remain accessible. Well-targeted and coordinated education and awareness campaigns on occupational activities and passive smoking by mothers during pregnancy could have a positive impact on improving the birth rate of underweight children.

Key words: Risk factors, low birth weight.

ABBREVIATIONS AND ACRONYMS

BCC: Behavior Change Communication ANC: Antenatal Consultation

EDS: Enquête Démographique et de Santé (Demographic and Health Survey)

EHS: Environnement d'Hygiène et Sécurité (Hygiene and Safety Environment)

FPN: Faible Poids de Naissance (Low Birth Weight)

Grs: Grams

HGR: Hôpital Général de Référence (General Reference Hospital) IC: Interval de Confiance

(Confidence Interval)

IEC: Information, Education, Communication Kgrs: Kilo grams

ITN: Insecticide-Treated Mosquito Net ODK: Open Data Kit

WHO: World Health Organization OR: Odds Ratio

ORa: Adjusted Odds Ration P: P-value

PB: Brachial Perimeter

CAR: Central African Republic

IUGR: Intrauterine growth retardation

DRC: Democratic Republic of Congo RVA: Régie des Voies Aériennes (Airways Authority)

SA: Week of amenorrhea

SNCC: Société Nationale des Chemins de fer du Congo (National Railway Company of Congo)
SP: Sulfadoxine Pyrimethamine

SPSS: Statistical Package for Social Sciences

IPT: Intermittent Preventive Treatment

UNICEF: United Nations Children's Fund

USA: United States for America WHO: World Health Organization

DEDICATION

To you, my very dear parents KALENGA KAMULETE François and TABU MUYUMBA, for your parental love, for giving me life and encouraging me to pursue my studies; here is the fruit of your sacrifices.

I dedicate this work to all of you.

François KALENGA LUHEMBWE

FOREWORD

As this work draws to a close, we would like to express our gratitude to all those without whose help this work would not have been possible.

To you Eternal God Almighty my shield, you have made me the tree that was abandoned and neglected by becoming the bearer of captivating and coveted fruit among so many others, thank you Heavenly Father.

Our gratitude goes straight to the Rector of the University of Kamina, Professor Paulin BANZA LENGE KIKWIKE, for his managerial spirit; to the Academic General Secretary of UNIKAM, Professor Georges KASONGO NGWELE, for coordinating teaching at UNIKAM.

To Professor Dr Michel KABAMBA NZAJI, supervisor and director of this work. I am happy and proud to have passed under your direction. You have my sincere gratitude. You have been able to accompany me despite my many demands. I admire your insistence on the importance of scientific evidence and your knowledge of maternal health.

To the Project Managers, Dr Ignace Bwana, Elie Kilolo Umba and Madame Marie Claire Balela, for guiding me without discouragement. Your sense of precision was an unwavering contribution. We are grateful for your trust.

Our thanks go to the entire School of Public Health management team for the smooth organization of teaching during this complicated academic year.

To all the teachers, supervisors and assistants at the School of Public Health, for providing us with the quality teaching that has made us what we are today.

To you, my dearest sweet Christelle Lenge, for your love, attachment and the courage you showed me during this difficult stage of my university studies.

To my dearest parents-in-law, MONGA KILUMBA Florentin and Chantal KALAMBA KABEYA, for their consideration, support and love.

To the Makonga family, we say thank you for your brotherhood. Your moral support has strengthened us greatly. A special thought to Madame Francine Makonga, Françoise Makonga, Murielle Makonga, Liliane Makonga and Vanella Makonga.

To our brothers and sisters, Patrice NSEGA, Trésor MWANAGOY, OKITO NGISI,

Emmanuel Kalenga, Esther Kalenga, Joelle Safi for their moral and social support.

To our fellow fighters, Giresse KABULO, Pierre NDAYA, Billy BULUNGA, Erick Nsensele, Lilly Mijibu, Sabine KADIATA, Lucie MBAYO, Mira MWEMA, Mireille KABANGA, for their advice.

François KALENGA LUHEMBWE

INTRODUCTION

0.1. Status of question

Low birth weight is a real public health problem for the 21ème century, as it is associated with high perinatal morbidity and mortality.

According to UNICEF (2004), low birth weight is defined as a birth weight strictly below 2500g, regardless of the term of pregnancy. It is a serious public health problem worldwide, particularly in low-income countries.

In the short and medium term, low birth weight predisposes to a number of pathologies, such as respiratory distress syndrome, infections, necrotic enterocolitis, hydrocephalus and mental retardation (WHO, 2005). It also increases the risk of certain conditions in adulthood, such as coronary heart disease, hypertension, type 2 diabetes and depression (Barker DJ & al., 2006).

Several obstetrical factors have been incriminated in the genesis of low birthweight at term, and their impact on infant morbidity and mortality is well recognized: the mother's young age, nutritional status prior to pregnancy, weight gain during pregnancy, parity, infectious and parasitic diseases, and the mother's lifestyle and work during pregnancy are the determinants frequently reported in the literature. Many authors have focused on the mother's risk factors, although socio-economic factors are insufficiently controlled for, and the potential for confusion between certain maternal variables (age, nutritional status, parity, etc.) is poorly taken into account. (Léger J., 2006).

According to the study conducted by Fatima B et al. (2013), on factors relating to low birth weight at the Sidi BA Obstetric Gynecology EHS (Western Algeria); the prevalence of LBW was estimated at 5.53%. The prevalence of LBW was found to be higher in primiparous women. This study confirmed the close association between low birth weight and maternal age between 20 and 34 years, gestational age below 37 weeks' gestation, and APGAR score<7, but also the role of other factors such as maternal pathologies, notably arterial hypertension, and gestational diabetes.

Another study conducted by Ghani H et al, (2015), on the etiology of low birth weight in the Islamic Federal Republic of the Comoros, had noted the following results: The average weight of newborns was 3351.72±561.64g, the frequency of LBW was estimated at 6%, the most dominant height was between 48-50 cm, the most dominant CP (head circumference) was between 34.5-35.6 cm, and 54% of newborns had a bip between 91.5-97.6

mm. The results of this study showed that maternal age, inter-gestational interval and parity did not correlate with newborn weight respectively (R=0.09, R=0.19, R= 0.12). On the other hand, mean newborn weight correlated with gestational age, uterine height, height, head circumference and bip, respectively (R= 0.46, R=0.51, R=0.55, R=0.62, R= 0.76).

Contrary to the results reported by Miaffo SL (2008), in his study on the risk factors and prognosis of low birth weight cases at the Yaoundé (Cameroon) gyneco-obstetric and pediatric hospital. The prevalence of LBW was estimated at 13.13%. The proportion of preterm hypotrophs was significantly higher than that of term hypotrophs, 85.6% versus 14.4% (p<0.001). Girls were in the majority, with 51.4% versus 48.6% of boys, but with no significant difference (p=0.892). The mother's age under 20, low level of education, primiparity, fewer than four antenatal visits, multiple pregnancies and maternal pathologies such as malaria, urogenital infections, arterial hypertension and anemia were the factors favoring the occurrence of FPN. Hospital mortality remained very high among LBW newborns, at 37.7%. The majority of deaths (79.04%) occurred in the early neonatal period. Very low birth weight, very high prematurity, poor Apgar score, extra-mural transfer, delivery in lower-level facilities and multiple pregnancies were identified as risk factors for mortality. Neonatal infections, prematurity, neonatal asphyxia and congenital malformations were the main causes of death. Length of hospital stay was longer in LBW infants, averaging 9.35 days versus 4.21 days in normal-weight newborns (Miaffo SL, 2008).

In a retrospective cohort study conducted in Malawi by Kalanda, risk factors for low birth weight in relation to the mother's anthropometric status were investigated. In this work 1571 pregnant women were followed and their anthropometric status was assessed by several measures. The following limits were used to define poor nutritional status: low brachial circumference (BP) (<23cm), short stature (<150 67 cm), underweight (<50 Kg) and low BMI (<18.5 kg/m²). In univariate analysis, mothers of short stature and low BP were significantly more likely to give birth to low-weight babies [OR=1.67; 1.14-2.45] (Kalanda, 2007).

Eloundou E (2016) for his part, in his study of risk factors aggravating neonatal morbidity and mortality at the Yaoundé Gyneco-Obstetric and Pediatric Hospital; The prevalence of FPN, was 9.1%. The majority of children born with FPN (75%) had experienced intrauterine growth retardation. Concerning prematurity, only the child's sex was significantly associated, showing a protective effect in boys. Conversely, boys were more at risk of LBW than girls.

Primiparous mothers and those with low anthropometric status were significantly more likely to give birth to LBW children, and this was mainly expressed by the IUGR mechanism, confirming that in developing countries IUGR is the major cause of LBW. Risk factor analysis using birth weight as a quantitative variable found similar results, and also showed an independent negative effect of the mother's short stature (<155cm). The researcher found no effect of placental malaria infection or maternal anemia. Children born with FPN, those with IUGR and those from nutritionally deficient mothers showed linear growth retardation. The author also demonstrated that LBW and the mother's low anthropometric status were significantly associated 8 with thinness. Malaria morbidity was not associated with staturo-weight development. Good dietary practices, as evidenced by a good IYCF score, were associated with correct corpulence, whereas they were paradoxically associated with linear growth retardation. Finally, in her cohort, boys grew less well than girls. Maternal nutritional deficiency (low anthropometric status or short stature) was implicated in the occurrence of FPN.

In order to identify obstetrical risk factors associated with low birth weight in rural Sahelian areas, Patrick Kabore et al conducted a cross-sectional study in central northern Burkina Faso, and enumerated 1013 newborns of a single pregnancy at term. After adjusting for socio-economic factors, primiparity (OR=2.8), gravidic vomiting (OR=3.4), rural work (OR=3.3), high workload during pregnancy (OR=1.6) and unassisted home delivery (OR=2.1) were the factors significantly associated with low birth weight, even though the number of prenatal consultations did not confer any preventive advantage against the occurrence of low birth weight. The study showed the need to redefine the content and procedures of pregnancy monitoring, including adequate management of gravidic vomiting, and to raise public awareness of the need to lighten the workload of pregnant women (Kabore P, et al., 2007).

Similar studies have also been carried out in the Democratic Republic of Congo, such as the one carried out in Lubumbashi by Makinko IP. et al. which revealed an FPN frequency of 13.0%. 18.7% were very premature. Extremely low birth weight represented 5.6% of cases, and very low birth weight 21.2%. The researchers observed that Apgar score at 5ème minutes (adjusted OR=2.4 [1.2-4.6]), resuscitation at birth (adjusted OR=3.9 [2.4-6.5]), early neonatal death (adjusted OR=10.3 [3.4-31.1]) were significantly associated with LBW. They also found that mortality rates decreased as birth weight and gestational age increased, with a statistically significant difference (p<0.0001) (Makinko IP. et al., 2016).

Also in Lubumbashi, according to the study conducted by Kabamba NM et al (2015) on the predictive model of low birth weight in Lubumbashi; passive smoking and the woman's unwillingness to become pregnant were significantly associated with the occurrence of low birth weight, with adjusted Odds Ratios of 4.28 (CI: 1.85 -9.93 at 95%) and 3.91 (CI: 2.20-6.95) respectively. Hospitalization and morbidity during pregnancy, and an insufficiently varied diet were also recognized as explanatory factors in the occurrence of low birth weight. However, the authors noted that a sufficient diet during pregnancy and a brachial circumference > 24 cm were protective factors for the occurrence of low birth weight, as their adjusted ORs were 0.13 (95% CI: 0.07-0.27) and 0.82 (CI: 0.73 -0.91) respectively.

In Kamina, a similar study was carried out in a semi-rural setting by Bwana KI. et al (2010), on risk factors for low birth weight in Kamina's semi-rural environment. This study reported an LBW prevalence of 14.3%. According to the same source, the factors associated with LBW were maternal age under 18 (OR=7.62, CI=3.46-16.8) and over 35 (OR=2.04;CI=0.91-4.46), primiparity (OR=2.48;CI=1.18-5.21) and non-attendance at prenatal consultations (OR=5.50;CI=2.00-15.03), prematurity with pregnancy less than 37 weeks of amenorrhea, multiple pregnancy (OR=30.94) and female sex of the newborn.

0.2. Issues

Low birth weight (LBW) is a major public health problem in both developed and developing countries, due to its scale and strong association with infant morbidity and mortality (WHO, 2010).

Every year, more than 20 million children are born weighing less than 2,500g. This represents 17% of all births in the developing world. Low-birth-weight infants are at risk of dying in the first months or years of life. Those who survive are at risk of having a deficient immune system and, later on, of contracting chronic diseases such as diabetes and heart disease more easily (Unicef 2017). According to the same source, low birth weight is responsible for the death of 9.1 million children every year worldwide, representing the leading cause of perinatal and infant mortality (UNICEF 2017).

The prevalence of LBW has fallen slightly, from 25 million in 1998 to almost 20 million in 2004, distributed as follows: 7.8 million in India alone; 5.3 million in Asia (excluding India); 4.3 million in Africa; 1.2 million in America and the Caribbean; and 1.1 million in China (UNICEF, 2004). In developed countries, the average is around 7%, half that of low-income countries (19%). Asia ranks first, followed by Africa (UNICEF, 2004).

In Europe, according to studies carried out by the World Health Organization, the percentage of low birthweight babies in industrialized regions is around 6.4%: 7% in France, 7% in Germany and 8% in Belgium. Northern Europe comes second: Denmark 5%, Norway 5%. Then Eastern Europe, with 5% in Ukraine, 6% in Russia and finally Southern Europe, with 8% in Portugal (UNICEF, 2006).

In the Americas, this percentage rises to 10%, with 2% and 8% respectively for Canada and the United States of America (UN, 2009).

Despite the efforts made, Africa still has the second-highest rate, with the incidence of low birthweight still higher than the standard set by the World Health Organization, i.e. below 10%. North Africa seems to be the most affected, with 15.3%. In West Africa, notably Senegal, a study conducted by the World Health Organization reveals a rate of 18%. In Central Africa, studies have revealed an incidence of 14% in Gabon, 14% in CAR, 17% for Chad, and 11% in Cameroon (EDS/Afrique, 2014).

In the DRC, the results obtained by Milabyo in Maniema during the 2003-2004 period showed that the proportion of low birthweight babies is no different overall from that in developing countries, and remains higher at 27% (Milabyo, 2006).

The Haut-Lomami province, our study area, has not escaped this alarming situation. According to recent statistics provided by Ignace Bwana Kangulu et al (2010), the prevalence of low birth weight was estimated at 14.3%. Faced with this constant concern about the problem of low birth weight, several questions came to mind, but we're going to focus on the main ones which are to know:

- What is the prevalence of low birth weight in the Kamina health zone?
- What are the risk factors for low birth weight in the Kamina health zone?

0.3. study objectives
03.1. Objective
The overall aim of this study is to help improve the health of the
mother-child relationship through appropriate health education.

03.2. Objectives
Specifically, this study aims to :

- To determine the frequency of low birth weight in the Kamina health zone;
- To determine the relationship between the child's birth weight and the various characteristics of the mothers and newborns involved in this study;
- Identify the various factors that may be associated with low birth weight in the Kamina health zone.

0.4. Hypothesis

There is a statistically significant association between low birth weight and socio-demographic characteristics, nutritional factors, socio-economic data, pathologies during pregnancy, toxic habits, distal determinants as well as newborn characteristics.

0.5. Choice and interest of subject

The choice of this topic is motivated by the fact that the prevalence of low birth weight is still high in the Democratic Republic of Congo, as in most developing countries, even though certain risk factors are entirely avoidable if they are well known. With this in mind, we decided to carry out a study on the risk factors for low birth weight, in order to determine what these factors are.

So, personally, this work will enable us to deepen our knowledge of low birth weight.

For the scientists, this work will constitute a very rich and necessary mirror of documentation which will help them to complete the investigations, and that this present work will be for them a model to follow and the results of this study can serve them to widen their ideas in this field.

Last but not least, this study will alert health and political authorities to the need to implement strategies and policies that will improve the health of the mother-child pair.

0.6. Methodology

This is a case-control study nested within a cross-sectional study that included live and non-living births registered at Kamina General Referral Hospital from December 2022 to July 2023. Data collection was based on a pre-established questionnaire enriched by an interview with the parturients concerned.

0.7. Delimitation

This work was carried out in the Democratic Republic of Congo, Haut-Lomami Province, in the town of Kamina and in the Kamina health zone, specifically at the Kamina general referral hospital, over a period running from December 2022 to July 2023.

0.8. Subdivision work

Apart from the introduction, conclusion and suggestions, this work is divided into two main parts: the first part deals with the theoretical approach and comprises one chapter including: Generalities on birth weight and the second part focuses on practical aspects and is made up of four chapters including: Presentation of the research environment; materials and methods; results and discussion of results.

Part I: Theoretical considerations

CHAPTER I. GENERAL INFORMATION ON LOW BIRTH WEIGHT
I.1. DEFINITION OF KEY CONCEPTS

- **Risk:** The possibility of an undesirable event occurring, the probability of a hazard occurring (Kermisch, 2011).

- **Risk factor:** Any attribute, characteristic or exposure of a subject that increases the likelihood of developing a disease or suffering an injury" (WHO, 2013).
- **Low birth weight:** Low birth weight is defined as a birth weight strictly below 2500g, regardless of the term of pregnancy. It is a serious public health problem worldwide, particularly in low-income countries (UNICEF, 2004).

I.2. NOTIONS ABOUT LOW BIRTH WEIGHT

The definition of low birth weight was adopted by the first World Health Assembly in 1948 as a birth weight less than or equal to 2500 grs. This definition was revised at the 29th World Health Conference in 1976, and a low-birth-weight child is now considered to be a newborn whose birth weight is strictly less than 2500 grs (Makki, 2002).

According to the value of birth weight, the World Health Organization (WHO) distinguishes three categories of underweight (WHO, 1975):
- Low birth weight: birth weight less than 2500 grs (up to 2499 grs included)
- Very low birth weight: less than 1500 grs (up to and including 1499 grs)
- Extremely low birth weight: less than 1000 grs (up to and including 999 grs).

Low birth weight results from two situations:
- premature birth, i.e. delivery before 37 completed weeks of amenorrhea (De Onis et al., 1998).

- intrauterine growth retardation (IUGR), i.e. delivery at term with a birth weight of less than 2,500 g, resulting in the birth of newborns who are small for their gestational age. In our study, they correspond to the group of newborns referred to as hypotrophic.

I.2.2. Factors associated with low birth weight

In the absence of precise information on the intrinsic causes of low birthweight, a wide range of information has been developed concerning risk factors, or factors whose presence in a woman is indicative of an increased likelihood of her giving birth to a low-birthweight child.

I.2.2.1.   The race

Black babies are twice as likely to weigh less than 2,500 grams at birth than white babies (Shiono, Klebanoff, Graubard, Berendes, & Rhoads, 1986). Some authors have suggested that the mother's age, rather than race, is responsible for this difference in birth weight between blacks and whites. Indeed, black mothers are often younger than white mothers at delivery. However, when the birth weights of mothers of different races of the same age are compared, the previously observed weight difference persists across all age groups (Starfield et al., 1991).

The same is true when other parameters, such as level of education, are taken into account. (Kessel, Kleinman, Koontz, Hogue, & Berendes, 1988) and (Collins, Derrick, Hilder, & Kempley, 1997), after correcting for biases in social conditions and demographic factors, have concluded that black individuals have a higher rate of fetal death, as well as a higher risk of giving birth to premature or intrauterine growth retarded infants. This racial disparity in birth weight is not due to socio-economic status. Race and socio-economic status have independent effects on the rate of low birth weight (Hulsey, Levkoff, & Alexander, 1991). This may suggest that genetic factors are involved in determining birth weight.

I.2.2.2.   Age

Adolescent mothers (aged under 20 at delivery) and those over 35 have the highest rates of low birth weight, compared with those aged between 20 and 30. However, other studies have shown that age alone does not explain low birth weight. Researchers do not yet agree that the mother's young age per se is a determining factor in prematurity or intrauterine growth retardation (Kramer, 1987). These teenage mothers often present other factors that increase the risk of delivering low-birth-weight babies: black race, low socio-economic level, short stature, low level of education, absence or inadequacy of prenatal health care. There is growing evidence that age is a social risk factor, not a biological one, except in the case of very young adolescents (Hediger, Scholl, Schall, & Krueger, 1997). Thus, the problems associated with teenage pregnancy are the result of psychosocial and economic circumstances, not biological ones (Turner, Grindstaff, & Phillips, 1990). When pregnant adolescents are prone to medical problems, lack of prenatal health care, malnutrition and the number of pregnancies, rather than age itself, may increase the risks (Wadhera & Millar, 1997).

I.2.2.3. Socio-economic status

Social factors and illness are undeniably linked (Liu et al., 2011). Low socio-economic status, expressed in terms of social class, income and education, is clearly associated with an increased risk of low-birth-weight delivery (Alexander & Korenbrot, 1995). The literature has shown that certain factors that increase the risk of low birthweight are found together in individuals of low socio-economic class. These include smoking, malnutrition, obstetric complications such as hypertension, pre-eclampsia, genital infections and limited access to antenatal care. Socioeconomic status represents the sum of several factors that individually increase the risk of low birth weight (Kogan MD, 1995). In Canada, low-birth-weight babies are 1.4 times more common in poor families than in wealthy ones. Studies in the USA and other countries have shown that the rate of low birthweight decreases with increasing socio-economic status. This is true when we take the following socio-economic factors into account These include the father's and/or mother's work, income and level of education (Alexander & Korenbrot, 1995).

It is not yet clear how socio-economic status determines birth weight. However, it is claimed that poverty, which is associated with reduced health care, malnutrition, low levels of education and an inadequate living environment, may be responsible for the increased risk (Klerman, 1991). Low socio-economic status is also strongly associated with other risk factors, such as women's behaviour and race. In addition to the consequences of poverty, there is also stress and anxiety caused by increased physical work, isolation, lack of social support, illness and frequency of childbirth (Chomitz, Lieberman, & Cheungl, 1992). (Sprague & Steward, 1998) conclude that the women most likely to give birth to low-weight children are also those with the fewest resources to care for them.

I.2.2.4.   Risks related to medical and obstetrical factors

These risks can be divided into two groups: those detectable before pregnancy, such as chronic illnesses in the mother, and those detectable only during pregnancy, such as infections of the placenta.

1.   *Pre- eclampsia*

Pre-eclampsia is a complication of pregnancy occurring during the third trimester. It is characterized by arterial hypertension and renal manifestations (proteinuria and edema) occurring in a previously intact kidney, disappearing without recurrence after delivery and causing serious maternal and fetal disorders. Studies carried out in the USA in the 1970s showed that 27% of intrauterine growth retardation may be due to arterial hypertension, pre-eclampsia and chronic vascular disease in pregnant women (Low & Galbraith, 1974). However, chronic hypertension without proteinuria does not correlate with poor pregnancy outcome (Carroli, Rooney, & Villar, 2001). Multiparous women with a history of pregnancy-induced hypertension are more likely to develop hypertension again than those without such a history. Women with a family history of obesity are more likely to develop pregnancy-induced hypertension. Nulliparous women are twice as likely to develop pregnancy-induced hypertension as multiparous women. Yet none of these factors, taken separately or in combination (neither socio-economic class nor dietary factors) can reliably predict who will develop pregnancy-induced hypertension(Rooney, 1992).

2.   *diabetes*

Diabetic mothers most often give birth to children who are too large for their gestational age, but the disease can also cause premature delivery or intrauterine growth retardation. It has been shown that inadequate control of a diabetic woman's pregnancy can contribute to the birth of children with low birth weight or congenital anomalies. Excellent control of these women from the very first weeks of pregnancy would reduce the risk of intra-uterine growth retardation (Lassmann-Vague V, Basdevant A, 1996).

3.   *Obstetrical history*

Information about the pregnant woman's previous pregnancies is of vital importance in predicting the birth weight of the unborn child. Studies in Norway, carried out between 1967 and 1973, have shown that the delivery of a low-birth-weight child in the first pregnancy is a powerful indicator of the chances of delivering a child of the same characteristics in the next pregnancy. Furthermore, the time interval between two pregnancies also affects low birthweight. The risk is very high for an interval of less than 6 months. It should be pointed out that a short interval between two pregnancies is not associated with the risk of delivering low-birth-weight babies, when the previous pregnancy ended in miscarriage (Bakketeig & Magnus, 1992).

4. Multiple pregnancies

Pregnancies resulting in the birth of twins, triplets or more are at risk of low birth weight. Twins are 11 times more likely to be born with a low birthweight than singletons. In fact, women with multiple pregnancies are more prone to hypertension and anemia (Papiernik & Keith, 1990).

5.   Genital infections

A multitude of infections are associated with premature birth and intrauterine growth retardation. Urinary tract infections and urogenital mycoplasma infections are the most common. The role of certain infectious agents in the birth of a low-birth-weight child has been established. For others, the association remains unclear. Most of these infections can be prevented or treated to reduce the risk of low birth weight (Kass EH, Mc Kuhn, 1981).

6.   Tropical diseases

Many common tropical diseases, such as malaria, schistosomiasis, intestinal helminthiasis and filariasis, have a major impact on reproductive health.

a.   malaria

Malaria infection during pregnancy is a major public health problem in all tropical and subtropical regions. In 1998, malaria cases were estimated at between 300 and 500 million, with 1,500,000 to 2,700,000 deaths, including 1,000,000 children under the age of five (Aubry P, 2003).

In most endemic areas, pregnant women are the main group of adults most vulnerable to the disease. The phenomenon has been studied mainly in sub-Saharan Africa, which accounts for 90% of the global burden of malaria-related morbidity and mortality (WHO, 2003). Every year, there are at least 30 million pregnancies among women living in malarious regions of Africa, most of whom reside in areas of relatively stable transmission. Moreover, estimates show that at least 24 million pregnant women are at risk from malaria in Africa every year (Steketee, Wirima, Slutsker, Heymann, & Breman, 1996). Indeed, pregnant women are at greater risk of developing malaria infection than non-pregnant women, since pregnancy reduces a woman's immune power. The fatality rate for cerebral malaria in pregnant women is around 50%.

During pregnancy, this burden is attributable to Plasmodium falciparum, the most common species in Africa. The effects of the other three human malaria parasites (P. vivax, P. malaria, P. ovale) are less obvious. According to estimates, malaria in Africa is responsible for 15% of maternal anemia, 35% of "avoidable" low birth weight and 5% of neonatal deaths (Wardlaw, 2004).

An association between placental infection by P. Falciparum and low birth weight has been demonstrated, and is more marked in primigravida babies (Matteelli, Caligaris, Castelli, & Carosi, 1997). From a pathophysiological point of view, placental infection is thought to reduce the transfer of nutrients and oxygen (Mireille, 2004). Malaria also contributes to low birth weight through anemia in the mother (Shulman, 1999). Maternal anemia due to malaria during pregnancy occurs through several mechanisms. Most notably, hemolysis occurs during the schizogonic cycle, and parasitized erythrocytes are destroyed. An autoimmune response is also involved in the destruction of non-parasitized erythrocytes. A reduction in red blood cell production has also been demonstrated, due to a decrease in their precursors (Menendez, Fleming, & Alonso, 2000).

The symptoms and complications of malaria during pregnancy differ according to the intensity of transmission and the level of immunity acquired by the pregnant woman (Menendez, 1995). Although the two transmission contexts below are presented as two distinct epidemiological frameworks, in reality, the intensity of transmission and the level of immunity in pregnant women vary from one end of the spectrum to the other, since conditions in the same country are not necessarily identical (Bouvier et al., 1997):

- In areas of low malaria transmission, pregnant women have not acquired a high level of immunity and generally become ill when infected with *P. falciparum*. They are two to three times more likely to develop a serious illness as a result of malaria infection than non-pregnant women living in the same area. Maternal mortality can result either directly from malaria (severe form), or indirectly from severe malaria-related anemia. In addition, malaria infection is likely to cause a range of damaging effects: spontaneous abortion, neonatal death and low birthweight due to intra-uterine growth retardation.

- In areas of high and moderate malaria transmission, including most of sub-Saharan Africa, most women have developed sufficient immunity that, even during pregnancy, *P. falciparum* infection does not usually cause fever or other clinical symptoms. In these a r e a s , malaria infection is mainly characterized by the onset of secondary anemia and the presence of parasites in the placenta. The resulting nutritional deficiencies in the fetus contribute to low birth weight and are a major cause of very poor infant survival and development. In these areas of high malaria transmission, *P. falciparum* infection during pregnancy is thought to be responsible for 10,000 maternal deaths per year, 8-14% of low birth weight cases and 3-8% of infant deaths (Mireille, 2004).

To reduce the incidence of malaria infection among pregnant women and their babies, the WHO recommends a three-pronged integrated approach (Nadège & Elisha, 2004):

- Intermittent preventive treatment (IPT): all pregnant women are given at least two doses of preventive treatment with an effective antimalarial during regular antenatal visits. The safety, cost-effectiveness and efficacy of this approach have been verified. An evaluation of intermittent preventive treatment in Malawi showed that it was accompanied by a reduction in placental infections (from 32 to 23%).

%) and the number of cases of low birth weight (from 23% to 10%). It also revealed that 75% of all pregnant women would use this treatment if offered (RBM, 2001). Various drugs have been approved for the prevention of malaria in pregnant women (RBM, 2001). They include: chloroquine, laméfloquine, antifolates in combination with antifolinics. Currently, Sulfadoxine Pyrimethamine (SP) is the drug of first choice for this treatment. Prevention consists in administering a full therapeutic dose during the second and third trimesters, as part of a prenatal consultation.

- Insecticide-treated mosquito nets (ITNs): reduce both the number of malaria cases and the mortality rate among pregnant women and their children. A study of a high-transmission area in Kenya found that women who slept under an insecticide-treated net every night during pregnancy had four times fewer premature or low-birth-weight babies. The use of an insecticide-treated net also benefits infants who sleep with their mothers, by reducing their exposure to malaria (ter Kuile et al., 2003).Effective management of malaria attacks: in areas of low or intermittent transmission, pregnant women have little immunity to malaria, and are two to three times more likely than non-immune women to contract a severe form of the disease. In these regions, rapid treatment of pregnant women with fever or malaria is the main treatment strategy (WHO, 2003).

b. Other tropical diseases

Malnutrition or anaemia due to intestinal worms can make pregnancy difficult, and at the same time be aggravated by it. It is not uncommon for nutritional anaemia in women infested with intestinal worms to be diagnosed for the first time during pregnancy. Intestinal helminthiasis is caused by worms transmitted mainly through the ingestion of contaminated food. The three most important parasites are : Ascariasis lumbricoides, Trichuris trichura and hookworms. Some 250 million people are infested with Ascariasis lumbricoides, which kills 60,000 of them every year. Hookworms infect an estimated 1 billion people worldwide, including 44 million pregnant women. Prevalence rates vary from 10-20% in dry areas to over 80% in rainy and humid tropical rural areas (Steketee et al., 1996).

According to studies carried out in Nepal (pregnant women) and Zanzibar (non-pregnant women), eradicating hookworm infections in the study population could prevent 41% to 56% of moderate to severe anemias(Stoltzfus, Dreyfuss, Chwaya, & Albonico, 1997).In addition to intestinal worms, diarrheal diseases and respiratory infections are very common among pregnant women in tropical zones, and have a major impact on intrauterine growth retardation. These conditions can reduce birth weight by as much as 45 grams (Kramer, 1987).

7. The mother's nutritional factors

Prospective and retrospective studies now show that maternal malnutrition at conception and inadequate nutrition during pregnancy can lead to intrauterine growth retardation (Nadège & Elisha, 2004).

In poor countries, the major determinants of low birthweight due to intrauterine growth retardation are nutritional: inadequate nutritional status of the mother before conception, short stature and low weight (mainly due to malnutrition during childhood) and poor nutritional status during pregnancy (low weight gain during pregnancy due to inadequate food intake, quantitatively and/or qualitatively). Countries with a high rate of low birth weight also have a high percentage of chronically energy-deficient women and a large number of malnourished children (WHO, 1997).

The mother's nutrition during pregnancy is especially important. Indeed, low weight gain during pregnancy can account for 14% of low birth weights due to intrauterine growth retardation, and this rate can be as high as 18.5% in populations with a high prevalence of low maternal stature (Shetty PS, 1986). (Kramer, 1987) carried out a meta-analysis of nutrition-related weight gain during pregnancy. He found that in mothers whose initial weight was low, weight gain during pregnancy greatly reduced the risk of giving birth to a low-birth-weight child. Recent trials have shown that supplementation with zinc, folate and magnesium, as well as protein and energy during pregnancy, can prevent low birth weight (De Onis et al., 1998).

8.   *Alcohol*

Research into alcohol use during pregnancy is fraught with difficulties. A variety of criteria are used to define the concepts of alcoholism, excessive drinking and moderate drinking. In addition, it is often difficult to distinguish constant consumption of small amounts of alcohol from irregular but excessive consumption (Sprague & Steward, 1998). According to (Newman, 1986), children of heavy drinkers (two to four drinks a day) often have neonatal difficulties, including low birth weight. The effects of alcohol are probably proportional to the amount consumed (Windham, Fenster, Hopkins, & Swan, 1995). (Virji, 1991) found a weight difference of 120 grs between babies of moderate drinkers and those of non-drinkers. Women who drink large quantities of alcohol are more likely to give birth to children with fetal alcohol syndrome or other disabilities. Intrauterine growth retardation is one of the harmful consequences of this syndrome (Chomitz et al., 1992).

Furthermore, (Faden VB, Graubard BI, 1997) have reported a very high risk of low birthweight in children of alcohol-dependent mothers. Alcohol crosses the placenta without difficulty and reaches the fetus in concentrations equivalent to those present in the mother's blood. However, the harmful effects of alcohol may be felt earlier in the fetus than in the mother, where it is less perceptible, especially during the first half of pregnancy (Driscoll, Streissguth, & Riley, 1990). Even when it does not cause significant abnormalities associated with fetal alcohol syndrome, alcohol can have an impact on intrauterine growth. Placental dysfunction and direct intoxication are two of the many repercussions of alcohol use (Virji, 1991).

9. *Smoking*

Maternal smoking is the most indisputable preventable risk factor, including passive smoking (Rubin, Krasilnikoff, Leventhal, Weile, & Berget, 1986). Indeed, the link between smoking and low birthweight has been demonstrated in worldwide studies of over half a million births (Sprague & Steward, 1998). Smoking contributes to low birthweight by causing intrauterine growth retardation (two to three times greater risk in smokers) and, to a lesser extent, prematurity (1.2 to 1.5 times greater risk), according to (Mainous & Hueston, 1994), (Aaronson & Macnee, 1991) and (Wu Wen et al., 1990). In low-weight newborns, authors have shown that smoking causes a variation in birth weight of at least 150 to 200 grs(Kline, Stein, & Hutzler, 1987)and 153 grs(Frank, Mcnamee, Hannaford, & Kay, 1994). The adverse effects of smoking on newborn weight are proportional to the quantity of cigarettes smoked (Hebel, Fox, & Sexton, 1988). The risk of low birthweight increases with the number of cigarettes smoked during the last trimester, taking into account the duration of pregnancy (Lieberman, Gremy, Lang, & Cohen, 1994). Smoking during pregnancy may have greater consequences for older women (Backe, 1993).

The mechanism by which tobacco affects a child's well-being is not yet fully understood. Of the 4,000 products that make up tobacco, nicotine and carbon monoxide (which reduce oxygen concentrations carried in the blood) are known to chronically limit the supply of oxygen to the uterus and prevent the fetus from developing normally (Mainous & Hueston, 1994).

Petridou and colleagues (1990) suggest a direct link between smoking and reduced estrogen levels in the mother. As estrogen promotes fetal growth, its reduction during pregnancy would limit the baby's development. Finally, according to (Ellard, Johnstone, Prescott, Ji-Xian, & Jian-Hua, 1996), smokers gain less weight than non-smokers during pregnancy.

I.2.3. The consequences of low birth weight

Low birth weight is associated with increased morbidity, mortality, weakened immunity and poor development in newborns and children (Bukenya, Barnes, & Nwokolo, 1991). For children born at term weighing between 2000 and 2500 grs, the risk of neonatal death is four times higher than for those weighing between 2500 and 3000 grs, and ten times higher than for children weighing between 3000 and 3500 grs at birth. In poor countries with a high percentage of neonatal deaths, intrauterine growth retardation is the major cause. Although the association between low birthweight and increased infant mortality is strong only in the early neonatal period, it extends beyond this period (Ashworth, 1998). What's more, low birthweight increases the risk of diarrhea and pneumonia in the children concerned for several months, especially in poor countries.

This risk is two to three times higher than for children of normal birth weight (Fonseca et al., 1996). Birth weight is an important predictor of weight and height later in life. Indeed, children born with intrauterine growth retardation fail to reach normal weight and height during childhood (Mason JB, Hunt J, 1999). Between the ages of 17 and 19, children born with low birth weight due to intrauterine growth retardation weigh 5 kgrs less and measure 5 cm less than those with normal birth weight. These differences can be observed in both poor and developed countries (Albertsson-Wikland & Karlberg, 1994).

Studies evaluating the effects of intrauterine growth retardation on the development of mental functions in affected children have shown that these children are at high risk of neurological dysfunction, especially if they come from poor families. This condition is associated with behavioral problems (clumsiness, lack of attention) and poor school performance (Goldenberg, Hoffman, & Cliver, 1998).

In addition, several immune functions are impaired in children with intrauterine growth retardation. The extent of this phenomenon increases with the degree of fetal growth retardation. This abnormality in immune function is maintained throughout childhood (Cater J, 1994). Studies have shown that this situation persists into adulthood, with low concentrations of Immunoglobulin E resulting in reduced immunity and increased risk of infection (Godfrey et al., 1994).

There are clear associations between fetal growth retardation and blood pressure, non-insulin-dependent diabetes, cardiovascular disease and cancer in adulthood. Indeed, inadequate nutritional intake during the critical phases of pregnancy and early childhood increases the risk of chronic disease in adulthood (Popkin, 1998).

Part two: Practical considerations

CHAPTER II. MATERIALS AND METHOD

II.1. MATERIAL

II.1.1. Study framework
II.1.1.1. Geographical location

Kamina General Reference Hospital is located in the capital of Haut-Lomami province, in the Democratic Republic of Congo.

It is bounded on either side by :

- ➢ The airfield to the north, not far from the RVA district;
- ➢ The Kaniama road parallels the railroad line not far from district 14;
- ➢ The New Apostolic Church and SNCC clinic to the east;
- ➢ The Kimbanguiste church and its school in the west.

II.1.1.2. Capacity

The Kamina general referral hospital has a capacity of 120 beds, divided between the traditional departments (gynecology-obstetrics, surgery, internal medicine and pediatrics).

The maternity ward concerned by this study has a capacity of 27 beds, including 18 beds in the large common room, 3 beds in three private rooms (1 bed per room) and 6 beds in two shared rooms (3 beds per chapter).

II.1.1.3. Administrative organization

Even if some of the services listed below are no longer functional
The Kamina general referral hospital currently comprises four main sectors:

a)   Internal services
-       Internal medicine ;
-       Surgery ;
-       Pediatrics ;
-       Maternity ;
-       Emergency ;
-       Gynaecology and obstetrics ;

-       Isolation.

b)   Technical medical services

-       Operating room ;

-       Blood bank ;

-       Technical delivery room.

c)   Administrative services

-       Administrator ;

-       Secretariat ;

-       Reception.

d)   External services

-       Medical consultations ;

-       Laboratory;

-       Radiology ;

-       Pharmacy ;

-       Prenatal consultations

II.1.1.4.   Kindergarten human resources

11 nurses of different levels and studies are assigned to the maternity ward of HGR/Kamina. They break down as follows:

-       4 level A3 nurse midwives ;

-       2 midwife nurses level A2 ;

-       1 multi-skilled nurse level A1 and

-       4 matrons.

The hospital's 13 doctors, all general practitioners, work there on a rota established by the hospital's management.

management (duty and on-call).

II.1.1.5.   Patient attendance at the HGR/Kamina maternity ward

The HGR/Kamina maternity hospital is the city's largest and oldest referral maternity hospital. It receives all cases, both simple and complex, in the area. Its geographical location (almost in the center of the town of Kamina), the availability of qualified personnel, especially doctors and an operating theatre, make it one of the busiest maternity units in the town of Kamina.

It contains a PMI niche where pre- and post-natal consultations take place.

II.2. METHOD
II.2.1. Type and period of study
This is a case-control study nested within a cross-sectional study, covering mothers and children born during the period December 2022 to July 2023.

The cross-sectional study enabled us to determine the frequency of low birth weight and fetomaternal characteristics. The case-control study enabled us to determine the risk factors for low birth weight.

II.2.2. Study population and sample
The population concerned by this study consisted of all newborns alive during the period of our investigations, born of mono-fetal pregnancy and registered at the maternity ward of the Kamina general referral hospital.

II.2.3. Defining a case and a witness

A case was defined as any newborn whose birth weight was strictly less than 2500g, measured to the nearest 10 grams on a SECA mechanical baby scale. A control was defined as any newborn whose birth weight was greater than 2500g. Each case was matched at the same survey site with four newborns of the same sex and age (to within 24 hours) born at term and weighing 2500g or more.

II.2.4. Data collection technique
To collect the data, we used interviews backed up by a carefully designed, pre-established questionnaire. The questionnaire was administered at the maternity hospital in the mother's language (Swahili or French) 48 hours after delivery.

II.2.5. Data processing and analysis plan
Data were collected using the ODK geo-collect tool and analyzed using SPSS (Statistical Package for Social Sciences) software version 20.0. Descriptive and analytical statistical analyses were carried out successively. The Chi-Square (P) test was used to test for dependence between the FPN (dependent variable) and the other independent variables. The significance level was $P<0.05$. The Odds ratio (OR) and its 95% confidence interval (95% CI) were calculated to determine the association between the random variables.

Logistic regression using Wald's stepwise method was used to adjust associations between the occurrence of LBW (dependent variable) and sociodemographic variables, nutritional factors, socioeconomic data, pathologies during pregnancy, toxic habits and distal determinants (variables selected on the basis of the p < 0.2 criterion).

II.2.6. Selection criteria
- *Inclusion criteria*

For this study, we included two groups of children:

• For the case group, we included all newborns weighing < 2500g, admitted to and having stayed at HGR/Kamina during the recall period (study period).

• For the control group, we included all newborns weighing ≥ 2500g, admitted to and having stayed at HGR/Kamina during the recall period (study period).

- *Exclusion criteria*

All newborns admitted or not to the HGR/Kamina and discharged against medical advice were included in the study. Stillbirths and newborns whose mothers came from another town or refused to take part in the study were also excluded.

II.2.7. Selected variables
Dependent variable

-Birth weight

Independent variables

IV.1.1.   Mother's socio-demographic characteristics :
- Mother's age

- Marital status
- Religion
- Mother's instruction
- Mother's professional status
- Salaried activity

IV.1.2. Obstetrical history
- Gestité
- Parity
- Gestational age

IV.1.3. Treatment of the mother in the household, desire and follow-up of the fat girl

- Mother's treatment in the household
- Desire for the big one
- Pregnancy follow-up
- Mother's decision-making power
- Mother's contribution to household expenses

IV.1.4. prophylaxis
- Taking medication to prevent malaria during pregnancy
- Regular use of the net
- Tetanus vaccination during pregnancy

IV.1.5. maternal morbidity
- Disease
- Hospitalization of the mother during pregnancy

IV.1.6. Mother's toxic habit, living conditions, perception of eating habits
- Mother's passive smoking
- The habit of drawing water in the third trimester of pregnancy
- Working in the fields during pregnancy
- Perception of food quantity and quality

IV.1.7. Characteristics of newborn babies
- Type of pregnancy
- Delivery mode
- Gender
- Malformations
- Child development

II.2.8. Ethical considerations

Before taking anthropometric measurements and other study parameters, we took our time explaining the purpose of our study; to this end, we made it our duty to explain to each selected parturient that the results would be used for scientific purposes only. Oral informed consent was thus obtained. Participation in the study was therefore unrestricted. For reasons of respect for the personalities of all participants in this study, we have maintained anonymity.

II.2.9. Study limitations and difficulties encountered

The present study would have been more relevant if it had also investigated the outcomes of an LBW child. It would still be useful to repeat other large-scale studies with larger sample sizes (city, province, etc.).

Throughout our study we came up against the following difficulties:

-	Insufficient financial resources and the support of parents and third parties enabled us to overcome this difficulty.

-	Untimely power cuts during work preparation; to get around this difficulty, we had to look for a place where there was a generator.

-	Insufficient data in some women's ANC follow-up sheets, making it difficult to assess their weight trends during pregnancy; we were therefore obliged to eliminate the variable weight trends during pregnancy from our study.

-	The absence of certain elements relating to newborns on the birth records (APGAR); we were obliged to prune the APGAR variable.

-	Some women refused to answer the questions; to get around this difficulty, we were obliged to give several explanations in order to convince them; if the refusal remained persistent, we were obliged to exclude them from the study;

CHAPTER III. RESULTS

III.1. Univariate analysis

III.1. Frequency of low birth weight

Birth weight	Numbers	Percentage
<2500g	19	14,28
≥2500g	114	85,71
Total 133		**100,0**

The results of this study show that out of a total of 133 births registered at the Kamina General Referral Hospital from December 2022 to July 2023, 19 low birth weight births were recorded, representing a frequency of 14.28%.

III.1.1. Mother's socio-demographic characteristics

Table II. Distribution of cases according to mother's age, marital status, religion, mother's education; mother's professional status and salaried activity

Mother's socio-demographic characteristics	Number (n=19)	Percentage
Mother's age		
<20 and >35 years	8	42,1
20-35 years	11	57,9
Marital status		
Unmarried	7	36,8
Bride	12	63,2
Religion		
No	5	26,3
Christian	13	68,4
Muslim woman	1	5,3
Mother's instruction		
Uninstructed	15	78,9
Educated	4	21,1
Mother's professional status		
Inactive	15	78,9
Active	4	21,1
Salaried activity		
No	16	84,2
Yes	3	15,8

The study shows that most of the mothers of FNP children (58.9%) are aged between 20 and 35; 63.2% of them are married; 68.4% are Christians; 78.9% are uneducated; 78.9% are professionally inactive and 84.2% are not salaried.

III.1.2. Obstetrical history

Table III. Distribution of cases by gestia, parity and gestational age

Obstetrical history	Number (n=19)	Percentage
Gestité		
Primigeste	7	36,8
Multigeste	12	63,2
Parity		
Primimare	8	42,1
Multipare	11	57,9
Gestational age		
$\leq$37 SA	14	73,7
>37 SA	5	26,3

This table shows that the majority of mothers of LBW children (63.2%) are multigestational; 57.9% are multiparous and 73.7% had a preterm birth.

III.1.3. Treatment of the mother in the household, desire and follow-up of the fat girl

Table IV. Distribution of cases according to the mother's treatment in the household, desire and pregnancy follow-up

Parameters studied	Number (n=19)	Percentage
Mother's treatment in the household		
Wrong	11	57,9
Good	8	42,1
Desire for pregnancy		
No	13	68,4
Yes	6	31,6
Pregnancy follow-up		
No	5	26,3
Yes	14	73,7

The above table shows that 57.9% of the mothers of newborns born to LBW suffer abuse in the household; 68.4% did not want this pregnancy and 73.7% of their pregnancies were monitored.

III.1.4. prophylaxis

Table V. Distribution of cases according to use of medication to prevent malaria during pregnancy, regular use of mosquito nets and tetanus vaccination during pregnancy

Prophylaxis	Number (n=19)	Percentage
Taking medication to prevent malaria during pregnancy		
No	3	15,8
Yes	16	84,2
Regular use of mosquito nets during pregnancy		
No	11	57,9
Yes	8	42,1
Tetanus vaccination during pregnancy		
No	4	21,1
Yes	15	78,9

This table shows that 84.2% of mothers giving birth to an LBW baby took medication to prevent malaria during pregnancy; 57.9% did not regularly use mosquito nets during pregnancy and 78.9% were vaccinated against tetanus during pregnancy.

III.1.5. maternal morbidity

Table VI. Distribution of cases according to the mother's illness and hospitalization during the course of the pregnancy
pregnancy

Maternal morbidity	Number (n=19)	Percentage
Mother's illness during pregnancy		
Yes	17	89,5
No	2	10,5
Hospitalization of the mother during pregnancy		
Yes	14	73,7
No	5	26,3

The results of this table lead us to say that 89.5% of the mothers of LBW children had an illness during pregnancy; 73.7% were even hospitalized.

III.1.6. Mother's toxic habit, living conditions, perception of eating habits

Table VII. Distribution of cases according to mother's passive smoking, habit of drawing water in the third trimester of pregnancy, work in the fields during pregnancy, perception of food quantity and quality.

Parameters studied	Number (n=19)	Percentage
Mother's passive smoking		
Yes	16	84,2
No	3	15,8
The habit of drawing water in the third trimester of pregnancy		
Yes	15	78,9
No	4	21,1
Working in the fields during pregnancy		
Yes	14	73,7
No	5	26,3
Perception on quantity of food		
Insufficient	1	5,3
Sufficient	18	94,7
Perception on quality food		
Unsatisfactory	15	78,9
Satisfactory	4	21,1

The above table shows that the majority of mothers of children in the FNF, i.e. 84.2%, were passive smokers; 78.9% were in the habit of fetching water in the third trimester of pregnancy; 73.7% did field work; 94.7% declared that their diets were sufficient in quantity and 78.9% said that their diets were unsatisfactory in quality.

III.1.7. Characteristics of newborn babies

Table VIII. Distribution of cases according to type of pregnancy, mode of delivery sex, malformations and evolution of the child

Characteristics of newborn babies	Number (n=19)	Percentage
Types of pregnancy		
Twin	1	5,3
Monofetal	18	94,7
Delivery mode		
Cesarean section	3	15,8
Low track	16	84,2
Gender		
Female	2	10,5
Male	17	89,5
Malformations		
Yes	1	5,3
No	18	94,7
Child development		
Deceased	1	5,3
Vivant	18	94,7

With regard to the characteristics of the newborn, this table shows that 94.7% of the mothers of LBW children had a monofetal delivery; 89.5% gave birth vaginally. The majority of FPN children (89.5%) were male; 94.7% had no malformations and 94.7% were alive at the time of our survey.

III.1.8. Bivariate analysis

Table IX. Relationship between FPN and mother's age, marital status and mother's religion

Features socio-demographic	*Case*	*Witnesses*	OR [IC95%]	P
Mother's age	n= 19	n=76		
<20 and >35 years	8 (42,1%)	21 (27,6%)	1,905 [0,673-5,390]	0,220
20-35 years	11 (57,9%)	55 (72,4%)		
Marital status				
Single	7 (36,8%)	17 (22,4%)	2,025 [0,690-5,944]	0,194
Bride	12 (63,2%)	59 (77,6%)		
Religion				
No	5 (26,3%)	11 (14,5%)	1,818[0,537-6,154]	0,332
Christian	13 (68,4%)	52 (68,4%)	1	
Muslim woman	1 (5,3%)	13 (17,1%)	0,307[0,036-270]	0,253

The table shows that mother's age (OR=1.905 [0.673-5.390]; p=0.22), marital status (OR=2.025 [0.690-5.944]; p=0.19) and mother's religion (OR=1.818 [0.537-6.154]; p=0.33) have a non-significant association with low birth weight.

Table X. Relationship between FPN and mother's education; professional status of mother and salaried activity

Features socio-demographic	Cases	Controls	OR [IC95%]	P
Mother's instruction	n= 19	n=76		
Uninstructed	15 (78,9%)	47 (61,8%)	2,314 [0,700-7,652]	0,161
Educated	4 (21,1%)	29 (38,2%)		
Mother's professional status				
Inactive	15 (78,9%)	41 (53,9%)	3,201 [0,972-10,540]	0,050
Active	4 (21,1%)	35 (46,1%)		
Salaried activity				
No	16 (84,2%)	61 (80,3%)	1,311 [0,338-5,091]	0,695
Yes	3 (15,8%)	15 (19,7%)		

The table shows that mother's education (OR=2.314 [0.700-7.652]; p=0.16), mother's professional status (OR=3.201 [0.972-10.540]; p=0.05) and mother's salaried activity (OR=1.311 [0.338-5.091]; p=0.69) were not significantly associated with LBW.

Table XI. Relationship between FPN and gestiture, parity and gestational age

Obstetrical history				
Cases Controls			OR [IC95%]	P
Gestité	n= 19	n=76		
Primigeste	7 (36,8%)	19 (25,0%)	1,750 [0,602-5,087]	0,300
Multigeste	12 (63,2%)	57 (75,0%)		
Parity				
Primimare	8 (42,1%)	19 (25,0%)	2,182 [0,765-6,224]	0,139
Multipare	11 (57,9%)	57 (75,0%)		
Gestational age				
≤37 SA	14 (73,7%)	56 (73,7%)	1,000 [0,319-3,132]	1,000
>37 SA	5 (26,3%)	20 (26,3%)		

In relation to obstetrical history; a non-significant association was found between gestia (OR=1.750 [.602-5.087]; p=0.3); parity (OR=2.182 [0.765-6.224]; p=0.1) and gestational age (OR=1.000 [0.319-3.132]; p=1.00) and FPN.

Table XII. Relationship between FPN and mother's decision-making power and mother's contribution to household expenses

Parameters studied

Mother's decision to spend her income					
Cases	*Controls*	OR [IC95%]	P n= 19	n=76	
personnel					
No	6 (31,6%)	22 (28,9%)	1,133 [0,382-3,359]	0,822	
Yes	13 (68,4%)	54 (71,1%)			
Mother's contribution to current household expenses					
No	9 (47,4%)	50 (65,8%)	0,468 [0,169-1,295]	0,139	
Yes	10 (52,6%)	26 (34,2%)			
Mother's decision on children's health					
No	6 (31,6%)	14 (18,4%)	2,044 [0,662-6,314]	0,208	
Yes	13 (68,4%)	62 (81,6%)			
Mother's decision on family planning					
No	6 (31,6%)	15 (19,7%)	1,877 [0,612-5,754]	0,266	
Yes	13 (68,4%)	61 (80,3%)			
Mother's decision on the day's meal					
No	3 (15,8%)	14 (18,4%)	0,830 [0,213-3,244]	0,789	
Yes	16 (84,2%)	62 (81,6%)			

A review of this table shows us that mother's decision on spending personal income (OR=1.133 [0.382-3.359]; p=0.82); mother's decision on children's health (OR=2.044 [0.662-6.314]; p=0.2); mother's decision on family planning (OR=1.877 [0.612-5.754]; p=0.26) had a statistically non-significant association with FPN.

Table XIII. Relationship between FPN and mother's treatment in the household and desire for pregnancy

Treatment of the mother in the household and desire for pregnancy	*Cases*	*Controls*	OR [IC95%]	P
Mother's treatment in the household	n= 19	n=76		
Wrong	11 (57,9%)	14 (18,4%)	6,089 [2,069-17,926]	<0,001
Good	8 (42,1%)	62 (81,6%)		
Mother's household considerations				
Wrong	8 (42,1%)	32 (42,1%)	1,000 [0,361-2,768]	1,000
Good	11 (57,9%)	44 (57,9%)		
Desire for pregnancy				
No	13 (68,4%)	9 (11,8%)	16,130 [4,89-53,104]	<0,001
Yes	6 (31,6%)	67 (88,2%)		

The above table shows that poor treatment of the mother in the household (OR=6.089 [2.069-17.926]; p=0.00) and unwanted pregnancy (OR=16.130 [4.899- 53.104]; p=0.00) were statistically associated with LBW.

Table XIV. Relationship between FPN and follow-up of last pregnancy and prophylaxis

Follow-up of last pregnancy and prophylaxis	Cases	Controls	OR [IC95%]	P
Pregnancy follow-up	n= 19	n=76		
No	5 (26,3%)	21 (27,6%)	0,935 [,300-2,919]	0,908
Yes	14 (73,7%)	55 (72,4%)		
Taking iron tablets or syrup during pregnancy				
No	3 (15,8%)	12 (15,8%)	1,000 [0,252-3,970]	1,000
Yes	16 (84,2%)	64 (84,2%)		
Taking medication to prevent malaria during pregnancy				
No	3 (15,8%)	10 (13,2%)	1,238[0,305-5,024]	0,765
Yes	16 (84,2%)	66 (86,8%)		
Regular use of the net during pregnancy				
No	11 (57,9%)	5 (6,6%)	19,525 [5,400-70,592]	0,000
Yes	8 (42,1%)	71 (93,4%)		
Tetanus vaccination during pregnancy				
No	4 (21,1%)	23 (30,3%)	0,614 [0,184-2,054]	0,426
Yes	15 (78,9%)	53 (69,7%)		

This table shows that not using a mosquito net regularly during pregnancy (OR=19.525 [5.400-70.592]; p=0.00) was associated with FPN. A non-statically significant association was found between taking iron tablets or syrup during pregnancy (OR=1.000 [0.252-3.970]; p=1.00); taking medication to prevent malaria during pregnancy (OR=1.238 [0.305-5.024]; p=0.76) and FPN.

Table XV. Relationship between LBW and rest during last pregnancy and maternal morbidity

Rest during last pregnancy and maternal morbidity

	Cases	Controls	OR [IC95%]	P
Stopping work during pregnancy	n= 19	n=76		
No	11 (57,9%)	22 (28,9%)	3,375 [1,197-9,519]	0,018
Yes	8 (42,1%)	54 (71,1%)		
Dispensing with household chores during pregnancy				
No	8 (42,1%)	24 (31,6%)	1,576 [0,562-4,419]	0,385
Yes	11 (57,9%)	52 (68,4%)		
Mother's illness during pregnancy				
Yes	17 (89,5%)	22 (28,9%)	20,864 [4,443-97,980]	0,000
No	2 (10,5%)	54 (71,1%)		
Hospitalization of the mother during pregnancy				
Yes	14 (73,7%)	10 (13,2%)	18,480 [5,463-62,509]	0,000
No	5 (26,3%)	66 (86,8%)		

In the light of this table, we say that there is a significant association between FPN and not stopping work during pregnancy, (OR=3.375 [1.197- 9.519]; p=0.01), the mother's illness (20.864 [4.443-97.980]; p=0.00) as well as the mother's hospitalization during pregnancy (OR=18.480 [5.463-62.509]; p=0.00).

Table XVI. Relationship between FPN and household socio-economic conditions

Socio-economic conditions household	Cases	Controls	OR [IC95%]	P
Household size	n= 19	n=76		
<5 people	13 (68,4%)	64 (84,2%)	0,406 [,129-1,279]	0,116
≥5 people	6 (31,6%)	12 (15,8%)		
Socioeconomic level				
Low	6	27	0,838 [,286-2,455]	0,747
High	13	49		

This table shows that household size (OR=0.406 [0.129- 1.279]; p=0.11) and household socio-economic level (OR=0.838 [0.286-2.455]; p=0.74) have no significant association with FPN.

Table XVII. Relationship between FPN and food consumption patterns Consumption

patterns food	Cases	*Controls*	OR [IC95%]	P
Number of meals	n= 19	n=76		
≤ 2 meals	12 (63,2%)	54 (71,1%)	0,698 [0,243-2,007]	0,504
> 2 meals	7 (36,8%)	22 (28,9%)		
Snacking during pregnancy				
No	8 (42,1%)	43 (56,6%)	0,558 [0,202-1,544]	0,258
Yes	11 (57,9%)	33 (43,4%)		
Clay consumption during pregnancy				
Yes	3 (15,8%)	8 (10,5%)	1,594 [0,380-6,689]	0,521
No	16 (84,2%)	68 (89,5%)		

A review of this table shows that FPN has a non-significant association with clay consumption during pregnancy (OR=1.594 [0.380- 6.689]; p=0.52).

Table XVIII. Relationship between FPN and activities during pregnancy and toxic habits

Activities during the pregnancy and toxic habits	Cases	Controls	OR [IC95%]	P
Mother's passive smoking	n= 19	n=76		
Yes	16 (84,2%)	26 (34,2%)	10,25 [2,737-38,434]	<0,001
No	3 (15,8%)	50 (65,8%)		
The habit of drawing water in the third trimester of pregnancy				
Yes	15 (78,9%)	67 (88,2%)	0,504 [0,137-1,856]	0,296
No	4 (21,1%)	9 (11,8%)		
Working in the fields during pregnancy				
Yes	14 (73,7%)	56 (73,7%)	1,000 [0,319-3,132]	1,000
No	5 (26,3%)	20 (26,3%)		

The results of this table show a statistically significant association between LBW and the mother's passive smoking (10.256 [2.737-38.434]; p=0.00). A non-significant association was found between field work during pregnancy (OR=1.000 [0.319-3.132]; p=1.00) and LBP.

Table XIX. Relationship between FPN and food perception

Perception of food

		Perception of quantity				
Cases	*Controls*	OR [IC95%]		P n= 19		n=76
Insufficient		1 (5,3%)	11 (14,5%)	0,328 [,040-2,715]		0,280
Sufficient		18 (94,7%)	65 (85,5%)			
Perception of quality						
Unsatisfactory		8 (42,1%)	28 (36,8%)	1,247 [,448-3,468]		0,672
Satisfactory		11 (57,9%)	48 (63,2%)			
Perception of variety						
A wide variety		15 (78,9%)	19 (25,0%)	11,250 [3,32-38,06]		0000
Not enough variety		4 (21,1%)	57 (75,0%)			

This table shows that there is a statistically significant association between FPN and the perception of a varied diet (OR=11.250 [3.32-38.06]; p=0.00).

Table XX. Relationship between FPN and newborn characteristics

Characteristics of newborn babies				
Cases *Controls*			OR [IC95%]	P
Type of pregnancy	n= 19	n=76		
Twin	1 (5,3%)	1 (1,3%)	4,167 [0,249-69,843]	0,284
Monofetal	18 (94,7%)	75 (98,7%)		
Delivery mode				
Cesarean section	3 (15,8%)	9 (11,8%)	1,396 [0,339-5,751]	0,643
Low track	16 (84,2%)	67 (88,2%)		
Gender				
Female	2 (10,5%)	19 (25,0%)	0,353 [0,075-1,670]	
Male	17 (89,5%)	57 (75,0%)		0,174
Malformations				
Yes	1 (5,3%)	1 (1,3%)	4,167 [0,249-69,843]	0,284
No	18 (94,7%)	75 (98,7%)		
Child development				
Deceased	1 (5,3%)	1 (1,3%)	4,167 [0,249-69,843]	0,284
Vivant	18 (94,7%)	75 (98,7%)		

This table shows that twin pregnancy (OR=4.167 [0.249-69.843] ; p=0.2); Caesarean delivery (OR=1.396 [0.339-5.751] ; p=0.6), malformative anomalies at birth (4.167 [0.249-69.843]; p=0.28); child outcome (OR=4.167 [0.249-69.843]; p=0.29) were not significantly associated with LBW.

III.1.9. Multivariate analysis using logistic regression

Table XXI. Logistic regression of different explanatory variables for low birth weight

Explanatory factors for low weight of birth	B	E.S.	Wald	pa	Exp(B)	IC for Exp(B) 95,0%	
						Lower r	Superior ur
No desire for pregnancy	3,488	1,161	9,023	0,003	32,736	3,361	318,829
Hospitalization during pregnancy	5,192	1,457	12,707	0,000	179,877	10,354	3124,88
Passive smoking by the mother during pregnancy	3,580	1,300	7,584	0,006	35,869	2,807	458,398
Constant	-5,104	1,524	11,222	0,001	,006		

Legend: B: regression coefficient; **S.E.**: standard error of regression coefficient; **Wald**: Wald test; **pa**: adjusted p-value; **Exp(B)**: adjusted Odds Ratio, **CI for Exp(B)**: confidence interval of Exp(B).

After adjustment by logistic regression, the risk factors for low birth weight were unwanted pregnancy (ORa=32.736; IC95%= [3.361-318.829]; pa=0.003) ; hospitalization during pregnancy (ORa=179.877; IC95%= [10.354- 10.354]; pa=0.00) and passive smoking by the mother during pregnancy (ORa=35.869; IC95%= [2.807-458.398]; pa=0.006).

CHAPTER IV. DISCUSSION

Today, low birth weight is a real public health problem, the frequency of which varies between developed and developing countries. Several studies have already been carried out on the subject in the USA, Europe, Asia, Africa, the DRC and even in the Haut-Lomami province, our research area.

IV.1. FPN frequency

The results of this study show that out of a total of 133 births recorded at the Kamina general referral hospital from December 2022 to July 2023, 19 low-weight births were registered, representing a frequency of 14.28%. Also in Kamina, a similar study was carried out in a semi-rural setting by Bwana KI et al (2010). This study reported an FPN prevalence of 14.3%. Similar studies have also been carried out in other towns in the Democratic Republic of Congo, such as the one conducted in Lubumbashi by Makinko IP et al. which revealed an FPN frequency of 13.0% (Makinko IP et al., 2016). The frequency of FPN in our study environment is close to that found in Cameroon by MIAFFO SL, where it was estimated at 13.13% (MIAFFO SL, 2008). Contrary to a study conducted in the Islamic Federal Republic of the Comoros by Ghani H et al. (2015), on the etiology of low birth weight in the Islamic Federal Republic of the Comoros, the frequency of LBW was estimated at 6%, much lower than that found in our study environment. This difference could be explained by the fact that our study was carried out in an urban-rural environment characterized by a low socio-economic level leading to food insecurity. This proves that FPN in our study environment constitutes a serious public health problem.

IV.2. Socio-demographic characteristics of mothers and LBW

Most mothers of LBW children (58.9%) are in the 20-35 age bracket; 63.2% are married; 68.4% are Christian; 78.9% are uneducated; 78.9% are professionally inactive and 84.2% are not employed. Maternal age (<20 and >35 years) and mother's religion had a non-significant association with low birth weight. Although Bwana KI et al found a significant association between LBW and maternal age under 18 (OR=7.62, CI=3.46-16.8) and over 35 (OR=2.04;CI=0.91-4.46) (Bwana KI et al., 2010); we are not the first to find a non-significant association between LBW and maternal age. Numerous other studies have highlighted the aspect that maternal age alone does not explain low birth weight. Following the example of Ghani H et al, (2015) in their study conducted in the Islamic Federal Republic of the Comoros, where maternal age did not correlate with newborn weight (R=0.09).

The mother's marital status (single) was not as significantly associated with LBW. Contrary to the findings of other researchers, celibacy could influence the child's birth weight status in one way or another, as the fact that the mother lives alone often means that she will be called upon to work hard to ensure her survival; this situation makes her more vulnerable to forced labor, field work or other physical activities that could have repercussions on her child's birth weight status. In a study conducted in Lubumbashi by Makinko IP et al. the mother's marital status was (adjusted OR=7.1 [1.2-28.6]) one of the maternal characteristics associated with LBW (Makinko IP et al., 2016).

IV.3. Obstetrical history and LBW

In relation to obstetrical history, a non-significant association was found between gestation (primigravida), parity (primipara) and gestational age (≤37 SA) and LBW. This observation can be explained by the fact that primigravidas and primiparas attend antenatal clinics more frequently (than multigestas and multiparas who believe themselves to be veterans), where they benefit from health education and adequate monitoring of their pregnancies. It could also be said that the more a woman conceives for the first time, the more her husband and relatives treat her like a princess; this situation can spare the mother-to-be from stress and anxiety, which in most cases are also factors favoring LBW and premature delivery. This observation is not in line with that reported by Kabore Patrick, et al. where primiparous women were (OR=2.8) times more likely to have an LBW baby (Kabore P, et al., 2007).

IV.4. Treatment of the mother in the household, desire pregnancy and FPN

Poor treatment of the mother in the household and unwanted pregnancy have been statistically associated with LBW. In relation to the relationship between LBW and unwanted pregnancy, several studies show that, nearly 80% of women who have unwanted pregnancy, live in a psychological depression that can have major consequences when it occurs during pregnancy (Unicef, 2016). Depressed pregnant women tend to eat less and sleep less. They also tend to be less involved in the medical monitoring of their pregnancy and less likely to comply with doctor's recommendations (O'Hara, 2009). In the most severe cases, depressed women are at risk of self-harm and have suicidal tendencies. Pregnant women with depression are more likely to have inadequate weight gain and feel more stressed than pregnant women with no or few depressive symptoms (Marcus, 2009). According to Dombrowski & Schatz; when left untreated, maternal depression is often associated with medical complications in the mother and/or newborn (increased caesarean sections, low birth weight or small head circumference, lower "Apgar" scores, prematurity, more frequent admissions to neonatology) (Dombrowski & Schatz, 2008). Some authors, such as Teixeira, Fisk, & Glover, note that depression causes maternal neuroendocrine and uterine blood pressure alterations, which contribute to premature birth, intrauterine growth retardation or pre-eclampsia (Teixeira, Fisk, & Glover, 1999).

IV.5. Prophylaxis and FPN

This study showed that non-regular use of a mosquito net during pregnancy was statistically significantly associated with LBW. This association can be explained by the fact that non-regular use of a mosquito net exposes the mother to malaria, which is one of the main risk factors for LBW. Studies have been carried out on this subject. According to Samuel N's analysis in Cameroon, the author found a significant association between LBW and non-use of mosquito nets (OR=6.2%; p<0.05); he also reported that the risk of having a low-birth-weight baby was 14.8 times higher in mothers who contracted malaria during pregnancy than in those who did not (Samuel N., 2019).

IV.6. Rest during last pregnancy and maternal morbidity

Based on this study, we can say that mothers who did not stop working during pregnancy run the risk of having an LBW baby. This is only to be expected, as various studies have shown that women who work during pregnancy are at risk of pregnancy complications. However, certain working conditions are recognized as a risk for pregnancy: standing work, carrying loads, working on industrial machinery and awkward working positions. A Dutch study which followed 4680 women between 2002 and 2006 showed that pregnant women who worked gave birth to babies of a lower weight (Snijder CA et al., 2006).

Similarly, mothers who have developed an illness during pregnancy are at risk of having a newborn with LBW; in the same vein, we say that maternal hospitalization during pregnancy exposes mothers to LBW 18.480 [5.463-62.509]; p=0.00. Previous studies have also shown a significant association between LBW and the mother's illness. MIAFFO SL (2008), in his study on the risk factors and prognosis of cases of low birth weight at the Yaoundé gyneco-obstetric and pediatric hospital (Cameroon). Maternal pathologies such as malaria and urogenital infections were significantly associated with LBW pa<0.1.

IV.7. Activities during pregnancy and passive smoking

The results of this study show that the mother's passive smoking exposes her 10.256 [2.737-38.434]; p=0.00 to LBW. A non-significant association was found between field work during pregnancy (OR=1.000 [0.319-3.132]; p=1.00) and LBW. Although the mechanism of action of tobacco on the child's well-being has not yet been established, it is known that the passage of nicotine and, specifically, its metabolite "nicotine" across the placental barrier has harmful effects on the fetus and unborn child through reduced oxygen intake. More studies have been carried out in various countries to investigate the contribution of smoking to low birth weight; according to Mainous & Hueston, (1994), Aaronson & Macnee, (1991) and Wu Wen et al (1990), smoking contributes to low birthweight by causing intra-uterine growth retardation (two to three times greater risk in smokers) and, to a variable extent, prematurity (1.2 to 1.5 times greater risk). In low-weight newborns, authors have demonstrated that smoking causes a variation in birth weight of at least 150 to 200 grs (Kline et al., 1987) and 153 grs (Frank et al., 1994). According to a recent study published by Thibert C. (2017), the more the mother smokes or stays next to a smoker, the more the baby suffers. The author's results show not only that a small exposure to tobacco alters birth weight, but also that this reduction is accentuated as the mother's smoking exposure during pregnancy increases. Thus, if the mother had smoked between 1 and 4 cigarettes or was a passive smoker, the birth weight loss was 228g. According to a Spanish study, more than half of non-smoking pregnant women are exposed to passive smoking. According to the author, the more non-smoking pregnant women are exposed to cigarettes, the higher the concentration of nicotine in their urine, and the greater the risk to the unborn child. Exposure to tobacco smoke increases the risk of fetal growth retardation, in neurological and cognitive development but also an increased risk of sudden death at birth (Juan U, 2018).

It has also been shown that the adverse effects of smoking on newborn weight are proportional to the number of cigarettes smoked (Hebel et al., 1988). The risk of low birthweight, given the duration of pregnancy, increases proportionally with the number of cigarettes smoked during the last trimester (Lieberman et al., 1994). Backe (1993) reported in 1993 that smoking during pregnancy could have greater consequences for older women.

CONCLUSION AND SUGGESTIONS

This case-control study investigated risk factors for low birthweight at the Kamina general referral hospital over the period December 2022 to July 2023. It was found that out of a total of 133 births registered at the Kamina general referral hospital from December 2019 to July 2020, 19 low birthweight births were recorded, representing a frequency of 14.28%.

Bivariate analysis showed a significant association between low birth weight and poor treatment of the mother in the household (OR=6.089 [2.069-17.926]; p=0.00); not wanting the pregnancy (OR=16.130 [4.899-53.104]; p=0.00); not using the mosquito net regularly during pregnancy (OR=19.525 [5.400-70.592]; p=0.00); not stopping work during pregnancy (OR=3.375 [1.197- 9.519]; p=0.01); illness during pregnancy (OR=20.864 [4.443-97.980]; p=0.00); mother's hospitalization during pregnancy (OR=18.480 [5.463-62.509]; p=0.00); mother's passive smoking during pregnancy (OR=10.256 [2.737-38.434]; p=0.00); perceived variety of food (OR=11.250 [3.325-38.069]; p=0.00).

However, the study showed that twin pregnancy (OR=4.167 [0.249- 69.843]; p=0.2), caesarean delivery (OR=1.396 [0.339-5.751]; p=0.6), malformative anomalies at birth (OR=4.167 [0.249-69.843]; p=0.28); child outcome (OR=4.167 [0.249-69.843]; p=0.29) were not significantly associated with LBW.

After Odds ratio adjustment, the risk factors for low birth weight were unintended pregnancy (ORa=32.736 [3.361-318.829]; pa=0.003); hospitalization during pregnancy (ORa=179.877 [10.354-10.354]; pa=0.00) and passive smoking by the mother during pregnancy (ORa=35.869 [2.807-458.398]; pa=0.006).

In view of all the above, we cannot conclude this work without suggestions which, if followed, could contribute to reducing the frequency of FPN in our study environment. These suggestions are addressed to political and administrative authorities, healthcare personnel, women and future researchers.

1. *The political and administrative authorities are asked to :*

- Improve the living conditions of the population in order to combat the low socio-economic level;
- Organize IEC/BCC activities on the importance of prenatal check-ups;
- Set up labor legislation (leave, smoking bans in the workplace, etc.) to protect

pregnant women's health;

\-   Support ongoing training for nursing staff.

2.   Healthcare personnel are reminded to :

\-   Make pregnant women aware of the risk factors for LBW,

\-   Educate mothers at ANC sessions about nutrition and prophylaxis for pregnant women, and healthy behaviors for pregnant women;

\-   Be able to diagnose at an early stage pathologies that could compromise the health of mother and fetus.

3.   Women and the general public are advised to :

\-   Avoid toxic exposure (passive and active smoking, alcoholism) during pregnancy

\-   Adopt family planning to avoid unwanted pregnancies;

\-   Have a correct and balanced diet, as its presence could have a positive impact on the birth weight of children;

\-   Stop working, especially in the third trimester of pregnancy

\-   Put into practice the measures proposed by health personnel on the healthy behaviours that a pregnant woman should adopt;

\-   Follow CPN as suggested by the health department;

\-   Regular use of the LLIN;

\-   Husbands should treat their wives well during pregnancy.

4.   Future researchers are advised to :

\-   To deepen this study by conducting others on a large scale with a large sample.

REFERENCES

Aaronson, L. S., & Macnee, C. L. (1991). Tobacco, alcohol, and caffeine use during pregnancy. *Journal of Obstetric, Gynecologic, and Neonatal Nursing: JOGNN / NAACOG, 18*(4), 279-287.

Backe, B. (1993). Maternal smoking and age. Effect on birthweight and risk for small-for-gestational age births. *Acta Obstetricia et Gynecologica Scandinavica, 72*(3), 172-176.

Barker DJ & Daum, R. S., Fridkin, S. K., Gorwitz, R. J. (2006). Adult consequences of fetal growth restriction. Clin Obstet Gynecol. 2006 Jun;49(2):270-83. [PubMed] [Google Scholar]

Bwana KI, Kilolo NU, Kabamba NM and Kalenga MK (2010). Risk factors for low birth weight in semi-rural Kamina, Democratic Republic of Congo [PubMed] [Google Scholar]

Cécile Thibert (2017). Passive smoking affects more than half of pregnant women

Dombrowski, M. P., & Schatz, M. (2008). ACOG practice bulletin: clinical management guidelines for obstetrician-gynecologists number 90, February 2008: asthma in pregnancy. *Obstetrics and Gynecology, 111*(2 Pt 1), 457-464.

Eloundou Estash (2006). Risk factors aggravating neonatal morbidity and mortality at the Yaoundé Gyneco-Obstetric and Pediatric Hospital. Faculty of Medicine and Biomedical Sciences, University of Yaoundé I. [**FubFacts| Google Scholar**].

Fatima Beddek and Dabis, F., Cousens, S., Some, A., Mertens (2013). Factors related to low birth weight at the EHS En Gynécologie Obstétrique de Sidi Bel Abbes (Ouest de L'Algérie). [**FubFacts| Google Scholar**].

Frank, P., Mcnamee, R., Hannaford, P. C., & Kay, C. R. (1994). Effect of changes in maternal smoking habits in early pregnancy on infant birth weight, 57-59.

Ghani H and Khang'Mate, F., Mwembo Tambwe A Nkoy (2015). Etiology of low birth weight in the Islamic Federal Republic of the Comoros. [FubFacts| **Google Scholar**].

Hebel, J. R., Fox, N. L., & Sexton, M. (1988). Dose-response of birth weight to various measures of maternal smoking during pregnancy. *Journal of Clinical Epidemiology, 41*(5),

483-489.

Juan urrekoetxea (2018). Tobacco smoke exposure and increased risk of fetal growth restriction.

Kabamba NM and Mukeng KC, Malonga KF, Kabyla KB, Luboya NO (2015). Predictive model of low birth weight in Lubumbashi. <u>Vol. 2, No. 2</u> [**RMSP**| **Google Scholar**].

Kabore Patrick, Philippe Donnen, M. D.-W. (2007). Obstetrical risk factors for low birthweight at term in rural Sahel. Santé Publique. 19:489-497. [PubMed] [Google Scholar]
Kalanda (2007). Risk factors for low birth weight in relation to maternal anthropometric status. MALAWI. [**FubFacts**| **Google Scholar**].

Kermisch Céline (2011). Le concept risque: De l'épistémologie à l'éthique, Lavoisier. ISBN 9782743013219.

Kline, J., Stein, Z., & Hutzler, M. (1987). alcohol and marijuana: Varying associations with birth weight, 44-51.

Léger J. (2006). L'enfant né petit pour l'âge gestationnel: sa croissance, son devenir. Médecine thérapeutique/ pédiatrie. 9(4):242-250. **PubMed**| **Google Scholar.**

Lieberman, E., Gremy, I., Lang, J. M., & Cohen, A. P. (1994). Low birthweight at term and the timing of fetal exposure to maternal smoking. *American Journal of Public Health*, *84*(7), 1127-1131.

Lynda MIAFFO SOKENG (2008). Risk factors and prognosis of cases of low birth weight colliges at the gyneco-obstetric and pediatric hospital of Yaoundé (Cameroon) [**PubFacts**| **Google Scholar**].

Mainous, A., & Hueston, W. J. (1994). Passive smoke and low birth weight: Evidence of a threshold effect, 875-878.

Marcus, S. M. (2009). Depression during pregnancy: rates, risks and consequences-- Motherisk Update 2008. The Canadian Journal of Clinical Pharmacology = Journal Canadien de Pharmacologie Clinique, 16(1), e15-e22.

Milabyo (2006). Prevalence of low birth weight in Maniema. DRC [Google Scholar]

O'Hara, M. W. (2009). Postpartum depression: What we know. *Journal of Clinical Psychology.*

WHO (2010). World report on low birthweight.
UN (2009). Low birth weight in America.

World Health Organization (2013). *Glossary.* Geneva: WHO Edition.

Paul Makinko Ilunga and Koontz, A. M., Hogue, C. J., & Berendes, (2016). Frequency and early neonatal prognosis of low birth weight in Lubumbashi, Democratic Republic of Congo [Google Scholar].

Samuel N. (2019). Association between malaria and low birth weight. Camerou..

Snijder CA and Leventhal, J. M., Weile, B., & Berget, A. (2006). Physically demanding work, fetal growth and the risk or adverse brith outcomes. The Generation R Study, Occupational Environmental. Medecin, 69:543-550.

Teixeira, J. M., Fisk, N. M., & Glover, V. (1999). Association between maternal anxiety in pregnancy and increased uterine artery resistance index: cohort based study. *BMJ (Clinical Research Ed.), 318*(7177), 153-157.

UNICEF (2004). United Nation Children's Fund. New York: UNICEF (2004). Low Birth.

UNICEF (2006). Low birth weight (Nutrition Policy Paper 18) [Google Scholar].

Unicef (2017). Multiple births: Trends and behaviours. Health Reports. (3):223-250 [PubMed] [Google Scholar]
WHO (2005). Definitions and recommendations. International statistical classification of diseases. 9th revision.
World Health Organization. Geneva: WHO (2005). Country, regional and global estimates. [Google Scholar].

Wu Wen, S., Goldenberg, R., Hoffman, H., Clivers, Davis, R., & Dubard, M. (1990). Smoking, maternal age, fetal growth, and gestational age at delivery, 53-58.

APPENDICES: Data collection form

I.   Identification number :

I.1.   Socio-demographic characteristics of the woman

1.   Age: / / / years

2.   Age of pregnancy :

3.   Marital status: 1.single 2.common-law or married monogamous 3.polygamous 4.widowed, divorced, separated / /.

4.   If polygamous, wife rank: / /

5.   Religion: 0. none 1.Muslim 2.Catholic 3.Protestant 4.other _______________________________

6.   Level of education: 0.None 1.Primary/Literacy 2.Secondary I 3.Secondary II 4.Higher education

7.   Professional status : 1.active 2.inactive / /

If employed: - salaried: 1.yes 2.no / /

Job type: 1.executive 2.owner/manager 3.self-employed 4.employee/skilled worker 5.labor and others / /.

8.   Size in cm :

9.   Brachial perimeter in cm :

I.2.   Socio-demographic characteristics of the husband

10.   Age: / / / years

11.   Level of education: 0.None 1.Primary/Literacy 2.Secondary I 3.Secondary II 4.Higher education

12.   Professional status: 1.Active Busy2   .Inactive / / If active busy: - Employed: 1.Yes 2.No / /

Job type: 1.executive 2.owner/manager 3.self-employed 4.employee/skilled worker 5.labor and others / /.

I.3.   Status of women

a.   Personal income

13.   Do you decide on your own how to spend your personal income? 1. yes 2. no 3. only in part / /

14. How much of your personal income is spent on running household expenses?

1. Nothing or very little 2.less than half 3. Half 4. more than half 5. all or almost all

/ /

b.   The woman's decision

15.   For each of the following situations, can you :

1. Decide alone 2.Participate in decision 3.Have no say

-       personal health / / - major household purchases / / - personal hygiene / / - personal health / / - personal health / / - personal health / / - personal health / / - personal health

-       children's health / / - day-to-day household purchases / /

-       family planning / / - visiting family, relatives, friends / /

-       meal of the day / /

c.   Ill-treatment

16.   Are you ever **abused** in your household? 1. yes 2. no

If YES, is it verbal abuse? 1. yes 2. no

17.   1. yes 2. no

18.   Generally speaking, in your household, would you say that you are respected/considered/treated in the following ways :

1. good 2.average3   .not very good

I.4. Follow-up of last pregnancy

19.   Did you want this pregnancy 1-Yes 2-No

20.   Presence of a logbook 1-Yes 2-No

Record ANC dates (or estimate months if no diary) and weight trends during pregnancy :

1ère CPN Date: /___________/____/____/ / / /, / / kg 2ème CPN Date: / /__________/____________/ ____________________________/ / / /, / / kg 3ème CPN Date : / /___________/____________/______ _______/ / / /, / / kg 4ème CPN Date : / /__/____________/____________/ / / /, / / kg 5ème ANC Date: / / / / /, / / / kg____________/____/____/ Female weight: / / / /, / / kg

I.5. Prophylaxis during last pregnancy

a.   Anemia :

21.   Did you take iron tablets or syrup during your pregnancy? 1-Yes 2-No If Yes: - from which

ANC? (note ANC number) / / - from which ANC?

22.   Did you take it regularly until the end of your pregnancy? 1-Yes 2-No / /.

If No: - estimated number of days covered / / / /

-        reason for interruption :

b.   Malaria :

23.   During your pregnancy, did you take any medication to prevent malaria? 1-Yes, 2-No
/ /

If yes: - which drug? 1-Fansidar 2- Chloroquine 3-Amodiaquine/Flavoquine 4-Quinine 5-Unknown 6-
Other / If other specify :

-        at what dosage? _______________________ What is the recommended dosage? 1- Yes, 2-No/ /
-        from which CPN? (note CPN number) / /
-        did you take them regularly until the end of your pregnancy? 1-Yes 2-No / /.
-        If no: - estimated number of days of protection / / / /
-        reason for interruption :

24.   Did you sleep under a mosquito net during your pregnancy? 1-Yes, 2-No / / If Yes: - was
this net impregnated? 1-Yes, 2-No / / - was this net impregnated?

25.   Avez-vous dormi régulièrement sous la moustiquaire pendant votre grossesse ? 1-Oui, 2-Non
Si Non : - nombre de mois de grossesse passés en dormant sous moustiquaire : / /
Has the rainy period been covered? 1-Yes, 2-No / /.

c.   Tetanus vaccine :

26.   Did you receive the tetanus vaccine during your last pregnancy? 1-Yes, 2-No
-        how many injections did you receive during the entire pregnancy? / /

d.   Rest: During your last pregnancy, did you :

27.   Have you stopped working? 1-Yes, 2-No, 8-No activity / / If yes, when did you start?
month ? / /

28.   Have you been exempted from household   chores? 1-Yes, 2-No, 8-No chores / / If yes,
from what month? / /

29.   Were you ill during your pregnancy? 1-Yes 2-No
If yes, what health problem(s) have you suffered from?

30.   Were you hospitalized during your pregnancy? 1-Yes 2-No If YES, what health problem(s) did you suffer from? Hypertension

Eclampsia Placenta previa Hemorrhage Malaria Diabetes Syphilis Anemia
HIV infection Urogenital infections Other (please specify) :

II. Gynaecological and obstetrical history

1.   At what age did you have your first pregnancy? / / / years
2.   Gestité / / / Parité / / How many abortions have you had? (spontaneous) / / /
3.   How many months are there between this child and his or her older brother or sister? / / /months
4.   History: 1.low birth weight YES NO 2. HTA YES NO

III. Household socio-economic conditions

5.   Composition: Total number of persons usually living in the household: / / /
6.   Housing: Roof: 1.tin/concrete 2.straw/straw 3.other : _________ Floor: 1.rammed earth/sand
2.rough cement 3.coated cement (tiles) Electricity in dwelling: 1.YES 2.NO / /
Drinking water: 1.tap in house 2.tap in yard 3.public fountain 4.other :
7.   Toilet type: 1.flush latrine 2.improved latrine 3.simple latrine 4.other :
Shared installation? : 1.YES 2. NO / /
8.   Assets owned: (indicate the number of each item included in the total package)
household)
-        Radios / / - Fridges / / If fridge, do you store your food in it? 1. YES 2.NO
-        Televisions / / - Other large appliances (freezer, ...) / /
-        Bicycles / / - Motorcycles / / - Cars (or other 4-wheelers) / / - Other
9.   Energy for cooking: 1.wood 2.charcoal 3.electricity 4.other : _____________________

III.   Food consumption patterns

10.   How many dishes/meals do you usually have a day / /?
11.   At what time of day? 1. Morning 2. Noon 4. Evening 8.other : _____________________
12.   How many of these dishes are eaten at home? / /
13.   During your pregnancy, did you change the number of meals per day? 1. yes 2. no / /
14.   If yes, number of meals per day (in general) during each quarter:T1 : / / T2 : / / T3 : / /
15.   Do you usually eat outside your main meals (snacking)? 1. yes 2. no If yes, 1. on a regular
basis: number of times per week / / / / /.
2. on an occasional basis: number of times per month / / /.
16.   During your pregnancy, did you change your snacking behavior? 1. yes 2. no / / If yes,

indicate for each trimester: 1. more 2. the same 3. less 4. stop Same 3. less 4. stop T1 : / / T2 : / / T3 : /
/

17.   Did you use clay (regularly) during your pregnancy? 1. yes 2. no

18.   Are there people around you (at home, at work) who smoke regularly?

1. Yes 2.No

If yes, did they often smoke next to you during your pregnancy? 1. yes 2. no / /

19.   During your pregnancy, especially in the third trimester, are you in the habit of fetching
water?

1. Yes 2.no / / if yes how far from your home / /

20.   During your pregnancy, especially in the third trimester, do you usually go to work?

rural 1. yes 2.no / /

21.   How much money do you spend on food / / per day?

IV.   Knowledge/perceptions of food

22.   In terms of quantity, you would usually say that your diet is: 1. sufficient 2. insufficient / / If
what is the reason for this? 1. money 2.availability 4.diet 8.other :

23.   During your pregnancy, in terms of quantity, would you say that your diet was: 1. sufficient 2.
insufficient / /

If insufficient, what is the reason for this? 1. money 2.availability 4.diet 8.other :

24.   In terms of variety, you would usually say that your diet is: 1. rather very varied 2. rather not
varied

quite varied / /

If answer 2, what is the reason for this? 1. money 2.availability 3.diet 4.lack o f knowledge 5. other :

25.   During your pregnancy, in terms of variety, your diet was: 1. rather very varied 2. rather not
varied enough / /

If answer 2, what is the reason for this? 1. money 2.availability 4.diet 5.lack o f knowledge 6. other :

26.   For each of the following types of food, do you think you have :

Usually During Pregnancy
-       sugar 1.rather too much 2. Just right 3. Rather not enough / / / /
-       fat 1.rather too much 2. Just right 3. Rather not enough / / / /
-       salt 1.rather too much 2. Just right 3. Rather not enough / / / /
-       meats 1.rather too much 2. Just right 3. Rather not enough / / / /
-       fish 1.rather too much 2. Just right 3. Rather not enough / / / /
-       fruit/vegetables 1.rather too much 2. Just right 3. Rather not enough / / / /
-       milk/cheese 1.rather too much 2. Just right 3. Rather not enough / / / /

- caterpillars 1.rather too much 2. Just right 3. Rather not enough / / / /
- potatoes 1.rather too much 2. Just right 3. Rather not enough / / / /
- egg 1.rather too much 2. Just right 3. Rather not enough / / / /

V. Characteristics of newborn babies

27. Type of pregnancy: twin monofetal

28. Mode of delivery: vaginal delivery, caesarean section

29. Date: time: place :

30. APGAR: good depressed indeterminate

31. Measurements: birth weight (in grams): height (in cm) :

Cranial perimeter (in cm): thoracic perimeter (in cm): brachial perimeter (in cm) :

32. Gender: M   F

33. Malformations: present absent type (shape) :

34. Obvious immaturity: yes no

35. Examination on arrival: weight: temperature :

Coloration: blue   erythrosic pink Tone: hypotonia quadriflexion

Respiratory rhythm: eupneic poly or tachypneic

36. Breeding method :

Reception area: near the incubating mother

Feeding: artificial milk breast milk force-feeding suckling

37. Product received: vit $_{K1}$ antibiotic iron other vitamins (please specify) :

38. Evolution :   alive   deceased

If deceased: time: age: cause: **Name & surname of investigator: Date :**

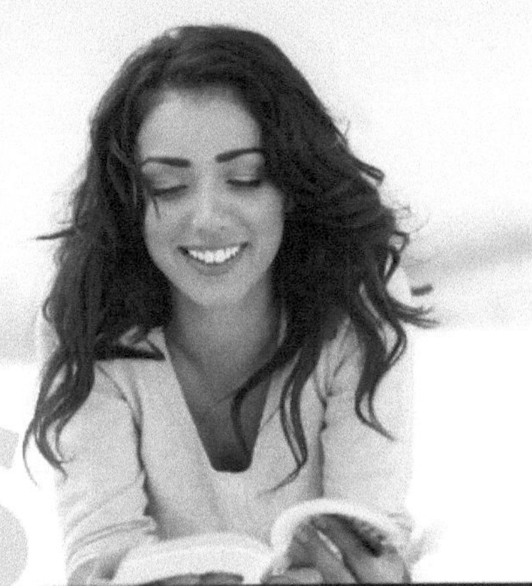

yes **I want** morebooks!

Buy your books fast and straightforward online - at one of world's fastest growing online book stores! Environmentally sound due to Print-on-Demand technologies.

Buy your books online at
www.morebooks.shop

Kaufen Sie Ihre Bücher schnell und unkompliziert online – auf einer der am schnellsten wachsenden Buchhandelsplattformen weltweit! Dank Print-On-Demand umwelt- und ressourcenschonend produziert.

Bücher schneller online kaufen
www.morebooks.shop

info@omniscriptum.com
www.omniscriptum.com

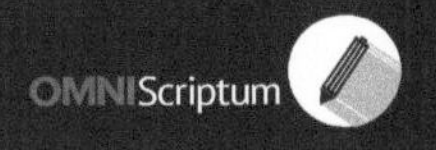

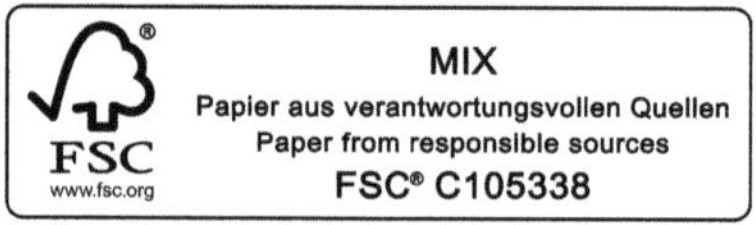

Printed by Books on Demand GmbH, Norderstedt / Germany